The Stay Younger, Look Hotter Guide to the Galaxy

"Healthy ways to look younger and feel hot again"

By
Harry J. Misner
http://www.HarryMisner.com

I0440229

<u>Disclaimer</u>

<u>LIMIT OF LIABILITY/DISCLAIMER OF WARRANTY</u>:

The Author makes no representations or warranties regarding the accuracy or completeness of the contents of this work. The advice, theories, and strategies listed in this book may NOT be suitable for all situations. Any use of this information in violation of any federal, state or local law is prohibited. All trademarks, trade names, services marks and logos referenced herein belong to their respective companies. Please consult your doctor or physician before starting any exercise or diet regiment.

- *Hold me now*

- *Touch me now*

- *I close my eyes and dream away*

- *I am still young but*

- *I crave for my youth*

- *Is it lost?*

$\mathcal{I}$ntroduction

This is the plight of every woman going through a middle age crisis. Can youth return? Can it be rediscovered? How can I keep my youthful appearance for a little bit longer? Do I look old? You don't look at me the way you used to look at me when I was younger. These are very familiar sounding questions. Chances are that these have been your own words.

Believe it or not, after health what most people grade as wealth is "youth". And I totally agree with them. I have my own reasons and they have their own, but the result is the same. Without youth you are err... err... OLD. With old age what come to your mind? Probably the first things that come to your mind are sickness, weakness and a fragile body with an equally fragile mind. Chances are you would shrug away the thought about you getting old. The fact remains unchanged that we all are getting older by the day.

No matter how hard you try to avoid this subject, you keep growing older and older till the time someone makes you realize it with very painful and matter of fact words.

Let me assure you this is not the end of it. God may not give you a second chance in life, but when it comes to youth, there is always a come around.

What I am saying here is not that I have found a magic spell that can turn you sixteen again, but what I can tell you is that you can retain and revive your youthfulness. It is all in your own hands.

What I want to tell you is that our life works on the principle of balance. The equilibrium of life means not to overdo one thing while neglecting another. This is a normal human tendency to do what we find convenient and to our likes, while leaving what we consider difficult and not to our taste.

*A*re *Y*ou *R*eady

Actually no one is ever ready for the silver haired era; some get it too soon, while others... they are just fortunate for the time being.

The first thing that has to be digested is the fact that you are not getting any younger. The second is your resolve to improve what you are today. So here is your bottom or base line marker. "YOURSELF ON THIS DAY".

Now what all you have to see are listed below:

⊕ Your weight

⊕ Your skin tone

⊕ Your vital statistics

The most important thing that you have to measure is your attitude towards yourself. Remember nobody will care about you if you are careless about yourself. So, be the first one to praise you, but don't forget to be honest. For that you will have to work very hard and earn it from nobody else but your own very self.

You're Weight

Just strip off to bare minimum and get on the bathroom scale. Note down the exact weight. This will become your start point for the days to come.

You're Skin Tone

Get a camera and get yourself photographed in daylight. A good close-up of your face without make up will tell you the real story. You don't have to show it to anyone but it will help you in judging your accomplishment later.

$\mathcal{Y}$ou're $\mathcal{V}$ital $\mathcal{S}$tatistics

Put on a one piece bathing suit and measure yourself in detail, without squeezing the measuring tape too tight.

- ⊕ Chest

- ⊕ Breast

- ⊕ Waist

- ⊕ Hips

- ⊕ Thighs

- ⊕ Calf

- ⊕ Arms

- ⊕ Wrist

These measurements will give you a fair idea as you go along with your new life.

The Golden Rules

For everything in this world there are some principles and rules to be followed. It doesn't matter if we like them or not but breaking these rules will only mean penalty for you.

In the years to come you will realize that making these rules part of your life will not just help you in maintaining a healthy life but will make you look and definitely feel a lot younger with an active and vibrant life style.

Rule #1 Sleep Well

Excess of everything is bad, but so is deficiency. In order to maintain a balanced and healthy life it is very important that every day we unplug ourselves from our daily hectic routine and put ourselves on a recharge. According to research our body actually replenishes itself during sleep.

An average human being can function normally for an extended period of time with sleep deprivation, but the cost is the overall wellbeing. Those who stay awake for longer hours and work very hard, their condition is pretty much visible from their appearance. Grey hair, dark circles around the eyes, fading complexion and uneven skin are a few things which are visible just from the appearance. Imagine all that is not visible. Here is a list of problems that can occur due to sleep deprivation.

⊕ Poor or lack of sleep is likely to cause alteration of hormones.

⊕ People who do not get enough *sleep* are more than twice as likely to die of heart disease.

⊕ Lack of sleep can cause Psychiatric disorders, including depression.

⊕ Poor sleeping habits can result in elevated blood pressure.

⊕ This is likely to cause diabetes even at a very young age.

⊕ Research has shown that people who continue to live with less sleep show all the signs of aging irrespective of their age, which include skin degeneration, poor metabolism, reduced absorption of carbohydrates and glucose, obesity and memory loss.

If you care about yourself, then these things are not to be taken lightly, as they are a matter of life and death, even most importantly a matter of keeping your youth.

This was just one side of the picture. The other extreme is excessive sleep. That too is not a healthy habit. As a matter of fact, excessive sleep really rusts you up. If you are in the habit of sleeping, then probably you wouldn't bother yourself to look younger in the first place and prefer to sleep the evening than to bother yourself to get dressed , look pretty and go out to have a great evening full of live and vigor. If that is how you feel, please stop reading any further and go take a long nap (AGAIN).

For those who care, this is a warning. Excessive sleep is as harmful as lack of sleep. The biggest problem attached to oversleeping is the attached lethargy that lingers on and prevents the person both physically and psychologically from leading an active life by causing a hormonal imbalance. The other factors caused by over sleep are listed below

⊕ Excessive sleep is the biggest reason behind obesity and weight gain, besides overeating.

⊕ Excessive sleep causes mental depression and lack of agility.

⊕ Excessive sleeping leads to muscle breakdown and reduced stamina.

Tips

Oversleeping once in a while is good, maybe on a weekend or during vacations, but when it becomes a habit it turns into an addiction. Housewives are really at a risk of getting into this addiction which is worse than any drug addiction.

There are a few ways to get rid of this problem, provided one realizes it and is willing to get over it.

In order to overcome it you'd have to be motivated and committed enough to do what it takes. Therefore I suggest that you start by writing down a few good reasons why you want to stop oversleeping. Read this list at least twice a day to strengthen your resolve.

Stop justifying yourself and stop making excuses for going to sleep early. Stop looking at sleep as a source of entertainment or relaxation. Instead, think about it as a waste of time. Something that you wish you didn't have to do.

Establish a routine and stick to it. Do your best to go to sleep at the same time every day. At least wake up at the same time, even on weekends. It may sound harsh, but it is essential till the time you gain control over your sleeping habits.

The first thing you should probably do is put the clock far away from bed, and commit to "not going back to bed after you turn off the alarm"!

Instead of focusing on the amount of sleep you're getting, start focusing on improving the quality of your sleep.

Here are a few tips for getting a good night's sleep.

⊕ Do not involve yourself with exhausting activities, like exercising, right before going to bed.

⊕ Steer clear of foods that are high in sugar like chocolate desserts and caffeinated drinks minutes before heading to sleep.

⊕ After working or studying, allow a couple of minutes of relaxation before you jump into bed.

⊕ Find suitable lighting for your room. Too much light can be distracting so you might want to turn it off for a restful sleep. On the other hand, some people can't sleep without the lights on. If this is the case, it would a good idea to have a study lamp on or anything that can be a source of dim light. Sleeping in bright light always cause a headache, as your eyes keep responding to light signals even during your sleep, and you end up un fresh.

⊕ Make sure that your room is noise-free by the time you hit the bed. Turn off all appliances, like TV or radio, which might keep you awake.

⊕ The temperature of the room is also of prime importance. If you have an air-conditioning unit in your room, make sure that you set it in your preferred temperature so you wouldn't have to wake up in the middle of the night to adjust the temperature because it's too warm or too cold.

⊕ Anxiety can also be a reason for sleeplessness. Try not to think of anything you should worry about before sleeping. If a soothing music can help you veer away from anxious thoughts, then you can turn on the radio to a soothing classic channel. Hard rock may not let you sleep and increase your anxiety.

Your physical condition could also dictate your sleeping habits. If you are not feeling well, you would obviously have a hard time getting some needed sleep too. Always consult your doctor if you notice any symptoms of any kind of ailment or disease. The topic of sleep is so vast and yet so little seems to be known about this great subject which is a daily part of our everyday lives. There are many interesting facts about sleep which you may not know about yet knowing these facts can immensely enhance your daily sleep.

The more you sleep the more energetic you feel. This couldn't be further from the truth as you don't need ten or eight hours of sleep in order to feel energetic and in fact contrary to standard beliefs, you only require five to six hours of sleep. Astonishing as it may sound, less sleep means you can perform better. In fact some of the world's greatest CEO's, entrepreneurs and scientists sleep only four hours a day and wake up full of energy and ready for yet another challenging day of work.

Do these people have a secret? Not really, here is another crazy fact about sleep. The more you sleep the more tired you feel. You may or may not have heard about this but in case you didn't know, over sleeping makes you lazy. This is pure common sense that if you sit in front of the TV all day doing nothing you're going to become a lazy couch potato. Sleep is the same thing if you over do it with passage of time, you will become lazier and lazier.

If you are someone who over sleeps, then try getting up early every morning and join the five O'clock club to see how this will affect your life. Believe me the results will leave you amazed at what you have achieved in that first single month in comparison to your previous year.

Rule #2 Eat Well

When I say eat well I definitely do not mean that you increase your diet. That will only increase your troubles. Eating well means that you eat what your body actually require.

A woman's body is different from a man's body (that is pretty much obvious) and so are its requirements. It is important to understand that a man does not require Iron and calcium as much in his diet as a woman requires it. There is a lot of wastage that needs to be recouped continuously.

Our life hangs in a balance; deficiency of a thing is as bad as the excess of it. It is therefore very important to keep your diet full of nutrients and minerals and yet maintain a balance in it without overdoing it.

Everything that nature has to offer to us has its benefits for us. What we have to see is that we select the right thing for ourselves. The list extends beyond count, but still a few are noted...

⊕ Carbohydrates

⊕ Fats

⊕ Proteins

⊕ Vitamins

⊕ Minerals

⊕ Salts

⊕ Water

⊕ fiber

These are just a few broad groups of nutrients that we require to maintain our bodies. Each and every one of them is important and the balance of our health depends upon its adequacy.

Carbohydrates

Carbohydrates are any of a large group of sugars, starches, cellulose and gums that are similar because they contain carbon, hydrogen and oxygen in similar proportions. Your body uses carbohydrates by converting them into glucose, a simple sugar, for fuel. Carbohydrates have 4 calories per gram.

Simple carbohydrates are also called simple sugars; these are found in processed and refined sugars including table sugar, honey and candy, and in fruits, vegetables, and milk products. Simple carbohydrates are more easily digested by the body than complex carbohydrates.

Complex carbohydrates, which are basically long chains of simple carbohydrates, are combinations of starch and fiber. Any food with starch contains complex carbohydrates: Examples are bread, cereals, pasta, rice, and starchy vegetables like potatoes.

Complex carbohydrates, because they contain fiber and some minerals, will do more for your body than simple carbohydrates.

However, when comparing sugars for health value, the sugar in an apple isn't any better or worse for you than honey, or table sugar for that matter. Your body digests it and uses it the same way regardless of where it came from.

Now here lies the problem, if you eat too much of any sugar, including the sugar found in dried fruits, you may develop cavities, and you could become obese. This would definitely make you a big turn off than a turn on.

Some Foods High in Carbohydrates

BREADS:					
ITEM	SERVING	CALOR.	FAT	FIBER	CARB.
IRISH SODA	1 slice	174	3g	1.5g	33.5g
PUMPKIN	1 slice	198.5	7.5g	n/a	30.5g
CORNBREAD, DRY MIX (Prepared)	1 piece (60oz)	188.5	6g	1.5g	29g
EGG BREAD	1 slice	115	2.5g	1g	19g
WHEAT, BRAN	1 slice	89.5	1g	1.5g	17g

DRY CEREALS:					
ITEM	SERVING	CALOR.	FAT	FIBER	CARB.
LOW FAT GRANOLA W/O RAISINS (K)	1 cup	427	6.5g	6.5g	88.5g
100& NATURAL, LOW FAT, CRISPY WHOLEGRAIN W/RAISINS (Q)	1 cup	389	5.5g	6g	80.5g
HEARTLAND NATURAL	1 cup	499	17.5g	7g	78.5g
SUN COUNTRY - GRANOLA W/ALMONDS (Q)	1 cup	532.5	20.5g	6g	76.5g
HEARTLAND NATURAL W/RAISINS	1 cup	467.5	15.5g	6g	76g
100% NATURAL W/RAISINS & DATES	1 cup	496	20.5g	7.5g	72.5g
BRAN BUDS (K)	1 cup	248.5	2g	36g	72g

PASTA:					
ITEM	SERVING	CALOR.	FAT	FIBER	CARB.
CORN, COOKED	1 cup	176.5	1g	6.5g	39g

RICE:					
ITEM	SERVING	CALOR.	FAT	FIBER	CARB.
WHITE, SHORT-GRAIN, COOKED	1 cup	242	0.5g	n/a	53.5g
WHITE, MED.-GRAIN, COOKED	1 cup	242	0.5g	0.5g	53g
BROWN, MED.-GRAIN, COOKED	1 cup	218.5	1.5g	3.5g	46g
BROWN, LONG-GRAIN, COOKED	1 cup	216.5	2g	3.5g	45g
WHITE, LONG-GRAIN, COOKED	1 cup	205.5	0.5g	0.5g	44.5g

Source: USDA - Nutrient Data Lab (Sept. 1996) - all data rounded to nearest 0.5

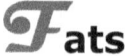ats

Fats are an amazing thing. Eating some fat is essential to health, but eating too much of the wrong kind can damage your heart.

Your brain is mainly made of fat. It's the fattiest organ in your body. Fatty foods taste good and are often very cheap. They are also available everywhere. But years of snacking on fatty foods can cause all sorts of health problems.

It can be very difficult to work out how much fat you're eating. Food labels are not always clear, and fatty take away foods don't say on the wrapper how much fat they contain.

Where there is a nutrition label, anything containing more than 20g of fat per 100g is a lot of fat. Try to cut back on these foods. Another thing you can do is... well, you're doing it right now. Learn about food so you can take control of what you eat.

But if you eat a lot of hard fats (like the ones in meat, butter and cheese), you're not doing your brain much good. The sorts of fat our brains need are found in fish and seafood, grains and seeds. All of these foods contain the type of fat, in the form of oil that is good for the brain.

Fats provide energy; gram for gram, fats is the most efficient source of food energy. Each gram of fat provides nine calories of energy for the body, compared with four calories per gram of carbohydrates and proteins.

Fats build healthy cells. Fats are a vital part of the membrane that surrounds each cell of the body. Without a healthy cell membrane, the rest of the cell couldn't function.

Fats build brains. Fat provides the structural components not only of cell membranes in the brain, but also of myelin, the fatty insulating sheath that surrounds each nerve fiber, enabling it to carry messages faster.

Fats help the body use vitamins. Vitamins A, D, E, and K are fat-soluble vitamins, meaning that the fat in foods helps the intestines absorb these vitamins into the body.

Fats make hormones. Fats are structural components of some of the most important substances in the body, including prostaglandins, hormone-like substances that regulate many of the body's functions. Fats regulate the production of sex hormones, which explains why some teenage girls who are too lean experience delayed pubertal development and amenorrhea.

Fat provides healthier skin. One of the more obvious signs of fatty acid deficiency is dry, flaky skin. In addition to giving skin its rounded appeal, the layer of fat just beneath the skin (called subcutaneous fat) acts as the body's own insulation to help regulate body temperature. Lean people tend to be more sensitive to cold; obese people tend to be more sensitive to warm weather.

Fat forms a protective cushion for your organs. Many of the vital organs, especially the kidneys, heart, and intestines are cushioned by fat that helps protect them from injury and hold them in place. (True, some of us "overprotect" our bodies.) As a tribute to the body's own protective wisdom, this protective fat is the last to be used up when the body's energy reserves are being tapped into.

Some scientists think that eating fish might have played a big role in helping human beings to develop the complex brains that we have now. They are getting more and more interested in the idea that if people ate more 'good fats' and less 'hard fats', then their brains might function better and they might end up cleverer. They also think that eating fish oils might help stop people getting depressed, because depression can be caused by the brain not working properly.

There is yet another controversy regarding fats. The good fats and the bad fats: To trim the confusing fat story into terms that help you make wise food choices, there are first three basic types of fats you need to understand: monounsaturated fats (MUFAs), polyunsaturated fats (PUFAs) and saturated fats (SATFAs) MUFAs and PUFAs are good fats; SATFAs are bad fats. How do you tell a good fat from a bad one? The good fats (MUFAs and PUFAs) are like oil. They flow through your arteries. The bad fats (SATFAs) act like sludge, sticking to the arteries. FA's are chemically known as fatty acids, but we call them fat.

What makes a good fat a healthy fat, and a bad fat an unhealthy one, has to do with the chemical structure condition of the fat known as saturation.

The fat molecule is composed mostly of hydrogen atoms attached to carbon atoms in a carbon chain. On this molecule there are open spaces, like parking spots. When all the available spots, or parking spaces, on the carbon atom are filled (i.e., saturated) with hydrogenated atoms, the fat is said to be saturated. If one or more places on the carbon are not filled with hydrogen, the fat is called unsaturated. A fat molecule with one empty space is called a monounsaturated fat, and is found in such foods as olive oil, canola oil, and nut oils. If two or more spots on the atom are empty, the fat is known as a poly-saturated fat, or, which is found primarily in vegetable oils and seafood.

At room temperature, some fats are solids (such as butter and lard) and some are liquids. The liquids are usually called oils. A saturated fat is solid at room temperature; an unsaturated fat is liquid at room temperature.

Whether or not fats help or harm the body depends upon their degree of saturation. Here's why. Unsaturated fat molecules (MUFAs and PUFAs) are a curved molecule with negative charges that repel each other so they don't stick together, resembling little bits of popcorn in a popper. Because these molecules don't stick together, they flow - both in the food and in the arteries. The molecules of a saturated fat are flat. They pile up like pages in a book and stick to each other. MUFAs and PUFAs are liquid at room temperature; SATFAs are solid at room temperature. Consider for a moment the fat molecules in your bloodstream. Do you want them to flow like oil or clump together like butter in your body? Choice is yours, burger with greasy fries or a fish salad.

Another interesting fat fact is that your body makes all the SATFAs it needs. You don't have to eat saturated fats. Is your body trying to tell you something? Yet, the body needs oiling. It needs MUFAs and PUFAs, which are why these fats are called essential fatty acids (EFAs). Your body can't live without them. While it can't live without MUFAs and PUFAs, we will live a lot longer if we eat less SATFAs.

Here are some commercial foods that are notoriously high in hydrogenated or saturated fat content:

⊕ Cookies

⊕ Airline snack foods

⊕ Some crackers

⊕ French fries

⊕ Pies

⊕ Shortening

⊕ Pot pies

⊕ Deep-fried burgers

⊕ Pretzels

⊕ Fried chicken

⊕ Doughnuts

⊕ Fried potatoes

⊕ Muffins

⊕ Corn chips

- ⊕ Stuffing's

- ⊕ Spoon-able dressing

- ⊕ Potato chips

- ⊕ Some peanut butters

- ⊕ Candy bars

- ⊕ Fast-food shakes

- ⊕ Nondairy creamer

- ⊕ Some cereals

- ⊕ Cakes

- ⊕ Margarine

- ⊕ Biscuits

*P*roteins

The fact remains that there is no life without protein. Protein is contained in every part of your body, the skin, muscles, hair, blood, body organs, eyes, even fingernails and bones. After water, protein is the most plentiful substance in your body. Proteins are composed of small units; these units are called amino acids (the building blocks of protein). There are 8 amino acids that we must get from foods these are called the essential amino acids. Most animal proteins contain all of the essential acids in sufficient amounts. The protein of cereals, most beans and vegetables may contain all essential amino acids, but the amounts in these plant foods is less than ideal, therefore making animal protein the most potent source.

Protein has a very important function in the body, that is, they rebuild the tissues which are damaged and help in building muscles. This action in turn burns stored fats. Proteins are also the main constituent of all hormones, which are responsible for almost every voluntary and involuntary action in our body, may it be directly or indirectly.

These actions range from feeling of hunger to digestion and from the feeling of arousal till delivery of a baby, the range is very wide. Lacks of Proteins not just causes physical problems but are also responsible for emotional instability and mood swings, especially in women. Imbalance in hormones plays havoc in a woman's body. The effects can range from mood swings to infertility and can also pose life threatening problems.

Foods of animal origin have the most protein. They are

⊕ Meat

⊕ Fish

⊕ Poultry

⊕ Eggs

⊕ Milk-based foods

⊕ Beans and legumes

These have a significant amount of protein. Think of dried beans (black beans, black-eyed peas, chickpeas, etc.), soybeans and soybean products and lentils, split peas and whole dried peas. Starches and vegetables have a small amount of protein, but it adds up over the course of a day.

Diets that contain no animal protein can cause a deficiency in those essential amino acids and are not recommended for anyone with growth needs, like, infants, children, teenagers, pregnant and lactating women and individuals suffering from wasting diseases, such as HIV/AIDS, or cancer. This has to be kept in mind when switching over to a vegetarian diet plan

$\mathcal{V}$itamins and $\mathcal{M}$inerals

Vitamins and minerals are required for the regulation of the body's metabolic functions, and are found naturally in the foods we eat. Many foods are fortified in order to provide additional nutrients, or to replace nutrients that may have been lost during the processing of the food. Most people are able to obtain satisfactory nutrition from the wide selection of foods available in the United States.

If a person is not able to eat a variety of foods from the basic food groups, then a vitamin and mineral supplement may be necessary. However, except for certain unusual health conditions, very few persons should need more than 100% of the Recommended Daily Allowance for any single nutrient. Large doses of vitamin and mineral supplements can be harmful.

Vitamins come in two varieties, fat soluble and water-soluble. Fat-soluble vitamins can be stored in the body for long periods of time, while excess amounts of water-soluble vitamins are excreted in the urine.

Here are a few facts about some of the vitamins and minerals that may give you an insight of what you are dealing with.

Vitamin A Is essentially required for new cell growth, healthy skin, hair, and tissues, and vision in dim light. The sources of getting it is from dark green and yellow vegetables and yellow fruits, such as broccoli spinach, turnip greens, carrots, squash, sweet potatoes, pumpkin, cantaloupe, and apricots, and in animal sources such as liver, milk, butter, cheese, and whole eggs.

Vitamin D actually promotes absorption and use of calcium and phosphate for healthy bones and teeth. We can get it from milk (fortified), cheese, whole eggs, liver, salmon, and fortified margarine. The skin has the capability of making its own vitamin D if exposed to enough sunlight on a regular basis.

Vitamin E protects red blood cells and helps prevent destruction of vitamin A and C. we can get Vitamin E from margarine and vegetable oil (made out of soybean, corn, sunflower, and cottonseed), wheat germ, and green leafy vegetables.

Vitamin K is very much necessary for normal blood clotting and synthesis of proteins found in plasma, bone, and kidneys. The main sources of Vitamin K are spinach, lettuce, kale, cabbage, cauliflower, wheat bran, organ meats, cereals, some fruits, meats, dairy products, eggs.

Vitamin C (Ascorbic acid) is an antioxidant vitamin C is needed for the formation of collagen to hold the cells together and for healthy teeth, gums and blood vessels. It improves iron absorption and resistance to infection. The sources available to us for getting Vitamin C are many fresh vegetables and fruits, such as broccoli, green and red peppers, collard greens, Brussels' sprouts, cauliflower, lemon, cabbage, pineapples, strawberries, citrus fruits.

Thiamin (B1) is required for energy metabolism and the proper function of the nervous system. The most common sources for ensuring it in your diet are whole grains, soybeans, peas, and liver, and kidney, lean cuts of pork, legumes, seeds, and nuts.

Riboflavin (B2) is a much needed component for energy metabolism, building tissue, and helps maintain good vision. It is sufficiently available in dairy products, lean meats, poultry, fish, grains, broccoli, turnip greens, asparagus, spinach, and enriched food products.

Niacin compliments Thiamin (B1) and Riboflavin (B2) in their functions which are for energy metabolism, proper digestion, and healthy nervous system. This too is available in lean meats, liver, poultry, milk, canned salmon, leafy green vegetables.

Vitamin B6 (Pyridoxine) is an essential component for cell growth the most confirmed sources of Vitamin B6 are; chicken, fish, pork, liver, kidney, whole grains, nuts, and legumes.

Folate (Folic Acid) promotes normal digestion; essential for development of red blood cells by ensuring proper absorption in the intestines. They are mostly found in liver, yeast, dark green leafy vegetables, legumes, and some fruits.

Vitamin B12 is required for building proteins in the body, red blood cells, and normal function of nervous tissue. It is abundantly present in liver, kidney, yogurt, dairy products, fish, clams, oysters, nonfat dry milk, salmon, and sardines.

Calcium is known for healthy bones and teeth, normal blood clotting, and nervous system functioning. It is found in dairy products, broccoli, cabbage, kale, tofu, sardines and salmon.

Iron is needed for the formation of hemoglobin, which carries oxygen from the lungs to the body cells. Its biggest sources are meats, eggs, dark green leafy vegetables, legumes, whole grains and enriched food products.

Phosphorus is essentially required for healthy bones and teeth, energy metabolism, and acid/base balance in the body. We can get Phosphorus from milk, grains, lean meats, food additives.

Magnesium is much needed for healthy bones and teeth, proper nervous system functioning, and energy metabolism. This again has its source in dairy products, meat, fish, poultry, green vegetables, legumes.

Zinc is required for cell reproduction, tissue growth and repair. We can find its sufficient quantity required for our dietary needs in meat, seafood, and liver, eggs, milk, whole-grain products.

Pantothenic Acid is needed for energy metabolism. Its sources are egg yolk, liver, kidney, yeast, broccoli, lean beef, skim milk, sweet potatoes, and molasses.

Copper is essential for synthesis of hemoglobin, proper iron metabolism, and maintenance of blood vessels. It is scarcely found in food groups other than seafood, nuts, legumes, green leafy vegetables.

Manganese is required for enzyme structure, is found in whole grain products, fruits and vegetables and tea.

$\mathcal{S}$alts

Salts are a life line for us, which are required in a very balanced quantity. The most of us know of them but rarely bother about its efficacy other than its taste

Sodium intake is recommended to be less than 3,000 milligrams daily. One teaspoon of table salt contains about 2,000 milligrams of sodium. The difference between "sodium" and "salt" can be confusing. Sodium is a mineral found in various foods including table salt (sodium chloride). Table salt is 40% sodium.

People with high blood pressure (hypertension) may be instructed by their doctor or dietitian to reduce sodium intake. High blood pressure can increase the risk of heart attack, stroke, or kidney disease. The body needs a small amount of sodium to help maintain normal blood pressure and normal function of muscles and nerves. High sodium intake can contribute to water retention.

Sodium is found in table salt, baking soda, monosodium glutamate (MSG), various seasonings, additives, condiments, meat, fish, poultry, dairy foods, eggs, smoked meats, olives, and pickled foods.

Potassium is essential for maintaining proper fluid balance, nerve impulse function, muscle function, cardiac (heart muscle) function

Sources: bananas, raisins, apricots, oranges, avocadoes, dates, cantaloupe, watermelon, prunes, broccoli, spinach, carrots, potato, sweet potato, winter squash, mushrooms, peas, lentils, dried beans, peanuts, milk, yogurt, lean meats.

*W*ater

Nobody can deny the importance of water and nobody can adequately emphasize enough on the importance of water. It not just keeps us from dying, but is a very important component for making us look good.

Normally we don't bother ourselves much about the intake and quality of water. Believe me these aspects play a vital role in our wellness overall and our appearance in particular.

Ideally, drinking water must taste good, be clear and odorless, and contain the right amount of mineral salts.

It should also be free of harmful substances, such heavy metals, nitrates, or bacterial or viral agents which may pose an infection risk.

Unfortunately, the water in many parts of the world is not of a good enough quality to drink. We must thank our lucky stars that we have it available in abundance and in good quality.

With the quality taken care of, what about the quantity? Are you drinking enough of it? Mostly women who work avoid drinking the right quantity of water just to avoid frequent visits to the ladies room. This is a very dangerous tendency. You are likely to dry up your body which is supposed to consist of 70% of water.

Deficiency of water is the biggest cause of urinary tract infections, and other skin problems.

What you should do is, start your day with a glass or two, maybe three glasses of water. This will help you regain what you have lost during your sleep. Then throughout the day frequently drink water. The more you drink, the more you conveniently you will remove toxins from your body, leaving behind the essentials and a well hydrated body looking gorgeous. Essentially one should drink 3-4 liters of water during winter season, and 6-8 liters during summers. If you are regularly working out don't forget to sip during your work out to avoid cramped muscles.

$\mathcal{F}$iber

Sources of fiber from highest to lowest are high fiber grain products, nuts, legumes (kidney, navy, black and pinto beans), vegetables, fruits, and refined grain products. They are basically of two types.

Soluble Fiber

These may help lower blood cholesterol by inhibiting digestion of fat and cholesterol; helps control blood sugar in people with diabetes. They are found in peas, beans, oats, barley, some fruits and vegetables (apples, oranges, carrots), and psyllium.

Insoluble Fiber

These helps prevent constipation, hemorrhoids, and diverticulitis. They are found in bran (wheat, oat, and rice), wheat germ, cauliflower, green beans, potatoes, celery.

Healthy Eating Tips

Reduce Fat and Cholesterol

⊕ Use skim or low-fat milk and cheese made from skim or low-fat milk
⊕ Cut back on the amount of fat you use in cooking
⊕ Use water-packed tuna instead of oil-packed
⊕ Choose lean cuts of meat
⊕ Trim visible fat from meat
⊕ Roast, bake, broil, or simmer meats and drain fat after cooking. Don't fry
⊕ Remove the skin of cooked poultry
⊕ Use smaller amounts of meat and stretch it by serving in casseroles with grains and vegetables
⊕ In a dip or sandwich filling, replace all or part of the mayonnaise with yogurt
⊕ Serve Canadian bacon instead of regular bacon
⊕ Use vegetable or peanut oils instead of solid shortening and use margarine instead of butter or lard
⊕ Try substituting egg whites in recipes calling for whole eggs

Control Calories

⊕ Avoid overeating. Eat only when hungry and just until you're full.

⊕ Moderation! Eat a variety of foods that you enjoy, but watch serving sizes.

⊕ Eat slowly and chew your food well. This allows you to realize you are full before you overeat.

⊕ Don't automatically have second helpings, unless it's a low-calorie vegetable or fruit.

⊕ Decrease your fat and sugar intake and your caloric intake will likely decrease.

⊕ Eat in a relaxed environment. It takes about 20 minutes after you begin eating for your mind to realize that you are full.

Reduce Sugar

⊕ Avoid high sugar foods - read labels for words like high fructose corn syrup, dextrose, sucrose

⊕ Use unsweetened canned fruit or fruit canned in its own juice.

⊕ Try using less sugar in your favorite recipes

Reduce Sodium

⊕ Decrease the amount of salt used while cooking
⊕ Taste foods before you add salt
⊕ Avoid high sodium foods - read sodium content on the labels
⊕ Drain and rinse canned vegetables

Increase Fiber

⊕ Eat whole grain breads, cereals, and pastas
⊕ Eat more raw fruits and vegetables
⊕ Nuts and seeds add fiber, but be aware of the additional calories
⊕ Add bran (1 to 3 tablespoons) into your daily diet. Mix it with cereals, casseroles, tuna salad, and muffins

Increase Calcium

⊕ Eat two or more servings of calcium-rich foods every day.
⊕ Examples: milk, cheese, yogurt, ice cream, cottage cheese, sardines or salmon (canned with bones), dried beans, tofu, broccoli.

Add Supplements to Your Diet

Normally we are unable to get all that is required from our diet, for the reason that we have our likes and dislikes. The end result is lack of one or more required nutrients. What can be done in this regards is to start taking a supplement that contains all the necessary ingredients.

There are several brands of supplements available in the market which has very high claims in fulfilling all sorts of dietary deficiencies. But there is one little problem with them, which is, that these supplements do really have those ingredients but they contain preservatives which does increase its shelf life, but at the same time kills the antioxidant qualities. This gives you a very marginal benefit of these supplements.

When buying a supplement choose something natural with very little amount of preservative. The best supplement available these days is the Aloe Vera. This is a naturally occurring tropical plant which is great for your skin and works miracles as it contains over three hundred different types of minerals and certain enzymes which are perfect for the user's digestive system, immune system and for the skin. Adding Aloe Vera or any other natural dietary supplement will definitely help you feel good and make you well nourished.

Rule #3 Exercises Well

Everything you do should be done in an organized manner for your own safety and for the sake of getting correct results. If by now you have decided to look good by eating correctly, you should also consider adding a fitness program in your routine.

People who exercise in general are less prone to diseases as compared to those who go on with it.

Getting Started

To begin from the beginning we have to consider a few basic things, which may not look important, but believe me these become the reasons for quitting. Most importantly they may affect the way you precede with your resolve.

Getting Medical Clearance to Exercise

Some may not consider it important but for your sake visit a doctor and get yourself examined before you start your fitness regime. Your doctor may be able to guide you in the correct direction keeping your present physical condition in view, especially, if you fall in one of the categories given below.

⊕ You've been diagnosed with heart problems, high blood pressure or other medical conditions

⊕ You've been sedentary for over a year

⊕ If you're over 65 and don't currently exercise

⊕ You're pregnant

⊕ You have diabetes

⊕ You ever experience chest pains, dizziness or fainting spells

⊕ You're recovering from an injury or illness

⊕ You have a diagnosed medical condition or illness

Use your best judgment and see your doctor if you have any questions about what you should be doing. Even if you don't have any problems, you may want to get a full check up before you start exercising, especially if it's been a long time since you've worked out.

If you have been inactive for a while, you may want to start with less strenuous activities such as walking or swimming at a comfortable pace. Beginning at a slow pace will allow you to become physically fit without straining your body. Once you are in better shape, you can gradually do more strenuous activity.

Proper Clothing and Footwear

Choosing the right fitness clothing and equipment is important for your exercise pleasure. Here are some general guidelines about deciding what to wear:

Think comfort. Shorts, tee shirts, tights, etc. you should wear whatever feels good to you. Test your clothes before you go to the gym (or wherever you're exercising) to make sure your clothes don't chafe, ride up, slide down or show more than you want.

Protect yourself. Wear light-colored clothes, a hat, plenty of sunscreen and sunglasses if you're exercising outdoors. You may also want to invest in clothes made of special wicking material such as Cool Max. This stuff keeps you cool and dry in the summer and warm in the winter...you don't need fancy fabrics, but it does make workouts more comfortable.

Wear the right shoes for your activity. For weight training and low impact activities consider a cross-training shoe, running or walking shoes. If you're going to be running, you'll want a running shoe so your feet will have plenty of support. Similarly, if you're participating in a sport such as basketball, football, etc. you'll want a sport-specific shoe so you don't hurt yourself.

Be safe. Make sure your clothes and shoes have reflective material on them if you're out and about at night.

Be very choosy about your workout socks. If they're too thick or thin you could get blisters which can ruin a good workout.

Choose clothes to fit your activity. If you're running or walking, a simple pair of shorts and tee shirt might be fine. If you're doing yoga or Pilates, you might choose more fitted clothing so you can move freely but stay covered.

There's no right and wrong when it comes to exercise clothes. It's whatever makes you feel good and keeps you comfortable.

Setting Your Goals

- ⊕ What do I want to accomplish with this exercise program?
- ⊕ Is my goal realistic and attainable?
- ⊕ Do I know how to reach my goal?
- ⊕ When do I want to reach my goal?
- ⊕ How will I reward myself when I reach my goal?

Keep In Mind That

- ⊕ The more weight you lose, the harder it will become to lose weight because the less weight your body has to move around, the fewer calories it will burn doing so.
- ⊕ The closer you get to your goal, the harder it will be to reach it, as a matter of fact, you may NEVER reach it (go talk to someone who's *still* trying to lose those last 5 pounds?).
- ⊕ The weight you can maintain may not be the weight you want to be.
- ⊕ Scale weight isn't always the best way to track progress. The scale won't tell you what you've lost and/or gained. Be sure to use other tools to track your progress, which I mentioned earlier.

⊕ Weight loss isn't the only goal you can have and may not even be the most motivating. Giving up the Weight Loss Obsession. This may be your first step to success.

It's helpful to know what you have to do before you get started. *Many people are surprised at the daily effort it takes to reach their goals.*

Once you know what you're doing and how you're doing it, you'll need some strategies for sticking with it:

⊕ Schedule your workouts
⊕ Set weekly goals and reward yourself each time you succeed
⊕ Work out with friends or family for added motivation
⊕ Recommit to your goals every day
⊕ Be prepared by always having your workout bag with you, bringing your lunch to work, etc.
⊕ Keep a food and workout journal to stay on track and measure your progress
⊕ Take your measurements regularly

Specific Health Benefits of Exercise

Work out not just help you to look great but it has definite health benefits too.

Heart Disease and Stroke

Daily physical activity can help prevent heart disease and stroke by strengthening your heart muscle, lowering your blood pressure, raising your high-density lipoprotein (HDL) levels (good cholesterol) and lowering low-density lipoprotein (LDL) levels (bad cholesterol), improving blood flow and increasing your heart's working capacity.

High Blood Pressure

Regular physical activity can reduce blood pressure in those with high blood pressure levels. Physical activity also reduces body fatness, which is associated with high blood pressure.

Noninsulin-Dependent Diabetes

By reducing body fatness, physical activity can help to prevent and control this type of diabetes.

Obesity

Physical activity helps to reduce body fat by building or preserving muscle mass and improving the body's ability to use calories. When physical activity is combined with proper nutrition, it can help control weight and prevent obesity, a major risk factor for many diseases.

Back Pain

By increasing muscle strength and endurance and improving flexibility and posture, regular exercise helps to prevent back pain.

Osteoporosis

Regular weight-bearing exercise promotes bone formation and may prevent many forms of bone loss associated with aging.

Psychological Effects

Regular physical activity can improve your mood and the way you feel about yourself. Researchers also have found that exercise is likely to reduce depression and anxiety and help you to better manage stress.

Setting Up Your Program

The next thing that comes up is, when to do it, I mean the exercise. The two good periods are the early morning and the evening. My favorite is the early morning routine which has its own advantages and is more beneficial.

⊕ You get to start you day earlier.

⊕ It tends to make you active through out the day.

⊕ The lethargic spell breaks.

⊕ No other commitment intervenes in this schedule and you get to continue it without a break.

⊕ You get to meet other people with the same routine which helps you increase and improve your circle of friends who are health conscious too.

Your exercise routine should start in a methodical sequence which I will discuss next in this chapter.

Warm up and cardio exercises

Each day your routine should commence with easy warm up routine. This puts you in gear to carry out other exercises. Remember, without proper warm up there are likely chances of getting yourself injured.

The correct way is to carry out light exercise for 5 – 10 minutes which will increase your heart rate in the initial 2-3 minutes and then you are required to maintain that heart rate for the next few minutes. This gives you the required warm up.

The cardio routine includes exercises which makes your heart rate to increase and then maintained at a particular rate for an extended period which should extend from 15 minutes to anywhere between 30 to 45 minutes.

The cardio exercises include all types of aerobic exercises, brisk walking and other forms of running styles ranging from jogging to sprinting. This depends upon your style, stamina existing state of fitness and what you can pull along for a long time as a routine.

For a beginner my advice to you is don't do it alone, join an aerobics class or take a friend with you to a park. Doing these exercises have an added benefit when done in the open. It makes you feel fresh and the air makes you feel less sweaty.

Strength Training

The routine continues after your warm up. Now it is time to build up your strength. It all depends up on your style and requirement. But let me tell you that strength training does involve basic muscle development and toning. For a man it is great to have well built muscles, but for a lady, no way. You should have well toned and firm muscles, but that's about all. You appear lady like, and that makes you hot enough. Men don't want you to become a lumberjack to get things heat up.

Strength training can be done with weights or machines or both. There are ways of doing it without the support of any machine or weights. This is the natural way, it takes longer than the modern techniques but it has its own advantages. If you have decided to join a health club or fitness center either try teaming up with a friend who has more experience than you or get yourself a trainer. This is a sure fire recipe for doing it right and not running away from the routine.

In the beginning, do it at the most 3 days a week and later increase a day when doing strength training. These breaks are essential as your body need rest as it was not used to this routine earlier. If you feel pain or discomfort in any single routine discontinue it for a couple of days. This will save you if there is any injury of a muscle caused by improper conduct of an exercise.

The most important thing is to do it right, not doing it more. So concentrate on doing it correctly instead of concentrating on increase your repetitions. Proper conduct of exercise has benefits in the direction of your aim, while improper conduct will only result in wastage of time and is likely to cause damage to your muscles.

If you are using weights, try it out initially with less weight. Increase the number of repetitions initially, instead of increasing the weight. Starting from 10 – 12 repetitions of a set per exercise increase gradually one repetition per day till you reach 16 repetitions. Then increase the weight and go back to 10 repetitions, repeating the same procedure again.

Flexibility

One thing is for sure, that is, we all need to stretch. Flexibility is a joint's ability to move through a full range of motion. Your muscles need to be flexible in order to allow your joints to move smoothly and to help avoid muscle tension and possible injury that may happen when your body is tight.

Stretching is one way to keep the body flexible, especially the muscles that are tight as a result of bad posture. Although stretching is typically the most overlooked part of an exercise routine, it's an important one and, for many of us, the best part of the workout.

Flexibility is an essential requirement of our body with the following benefits.

⊕ You'll improve your performance and reduce your risk of injury

⊕ You'll reduce muscle soreness and improve your posture

⊕ You'll help reduce lower back pain

⊕ You'll increase blood circulation and supply of nutrients to the tissues

⊕ You'll improve your muscle coordination

⊕ You'll enjoy exercise more and help reduce stress

It is very important to know how to Stretch. This will help you a long way in improving your posture and overall appearance. A person with a slouchy posture is a definite turn off. This is what you have to keep in mind when you start your flexibility work out.

⊕ Your best bet is to stretch after your strength workout when your muscles are warm and you're ready for a cool down. You don't have to stretch before your workout but, if you do, make sure you do it after the warm up. Stretching cold muscles can cause injury.

⊕ When doing static stretches, don't bounce. Hold a comfortable position until you feel a gentle pull on your muscle. It shouldn't hurt and bouncing could cause you to pull a muscle.

⊕ Try to hold each stretch for 15-30 seconds to get some long-term flexibility benefits.

⊕ You can also stretch between strength training sets and you may want to perform light stretches throughout the day to deal with tight shoulders, neck and lower back.

When you stretch after the workout, try to hit all the muscles you used, paying close attention to any chronically tight areas, especially your back and thighs.

$\mathcal{S}$etting $\mathcal{U}$p a $\mathcal{C}$omplete $\mathcal{P}$rogram

It is a requirement that you make a complete plan and then follow it religiously. To decide when to do what and when not to do what is a very important factor which needs to be deliberated upon.

If you are a beginner then, you should start slowly with a basic cardio program and a full body resistance training routine. You'll want to have recovery days to allow your body to rest and your muscles to heal from your new routine. A typical beginner program will include about 3 or so days of cardio and about 2 days of strength training. Below is a sample schedule which I have chalked out just to give you an idea of a typical week of workouts. But remember nothing gets started without a warm up.

- ⊕ Monday: 20 – 30 minutes cardio + stretching exercises.
- ⊕ Tuesday: Strength exercises + stretching.
- ⊕ Wednesday: 20 – 30 minutes cardio + stretching exercises.
- ⊕ Thursday: Rest or light stretching exercises.

- Friday: Strength exercises + stretching exercises.
- Saturday: 20 – 30 minutes cardio + stretching exercises.
- Sunday: Definitely rest.

Proper Nutrition

When you work out on a regular routine your body needs regular nourishment and proper nutrition to coup up with the body losses and repair work. Surprisingly eating helps reduce fats, but only the right type of stuff. You have to keep a vigilant eye on what you eat. Never exceed your intake calories beyond what you are burning.

Dietitians very strongly recommend that you eat smaller meals 5 or 6 times throughout the day to keep your blood sugar on a nice even level. Eating more frequently actually speeds up your metabolism. You never thought you'd have to eat to lose weight, did you? You have to ensure the following things

- Keep track of what you're eating, this means no more mindless munching! Keep a strict on our calorie intake.

⊕ Be aware of emotional eating or nibbling out of boredom. Find out what triggers this type of eating and keep yourself busy during those urges to munch. Keep your free time occupied in something useful or just fun. Remember, eating is not a fun pass time hobby.

⊕ Stay well hydrated. The more you dink the better you will feel. Often a feeling of hunger is actually your body telling you it's thirsty. Drink up!

⊕ Eat lots of fruits and veggies...the fiber will help you feel full and your body will thank for all the vitamins and minerals that will come as a bonus.

⊕ If you're starving, eat! When you wait too long, you may end up eating more food to satisfy that gnawing hunger.

⊙ What you need is a steady routine, starving does not fall in the routine category. So quit this habit, it will only harm you.

*M*aintaining *Y*our *E*xercise *P*rogram

Avoiding Plateaus

Plateaus occur exactly when you feel that your routine has now become stable and everything is going on just great. Actually this is the reason. Your body will adjust to any exercise program over a period of time, so you need to fool your body into continuing to progress by changing your program every six weeks or so. Not only should you change your cardio workouts, you should also change your strength training routines as well. This will keep your muscles confused so that they're constantly challenged. There are many ways to change your routines. Here are a few ways to fool your own system.

- ⊕ Changing the frequency (adding a day or subtracting a day of workouts)
- ⊕ Changing the intensity (adding more or less weight to your exercises, or working harder or easier on your cardio)
- ⊕ Changing the duration of time for exercising (if you usually walk for 20 minutes, try walking for 25 or 30 minutes)

⊕ Changing the type of activity (for strength training, changing the exercises, for cardio trying something completely new)

Keeping track of your workouts can help you determine when you need to change them. Use a calendar or a workout log and write down your workouts for six weeks. At the end of that time, sit down with your log and create a new routine by changing the routines.

When to Take a Break

Just as important we feel exercise to be, the requirement to rest is also no less important. Rest is required to recoup lost energy and regain vigor. Our body itself is the biggest alarm for this purpose. Listen to your body by keeping an eye on these tell tale signs of overexertion.

⊕ Insomnia
⊕ Achiness or pain in the muscles and/or joints
⊕ Fatigue
⊕ Headaches
⊕ Elevated morning pulse

- Sudden inability to complete workouts
- Feeling unmotivated and lacking energy
- Increased susceptibility to colds, sore throats and other illnesses
- Loss in appetite
- Decrease in performance

If any of these signs appear, it means that you have over trained yourself and it is time for a break.

Your break period is also dictated by your body, which can range between a few days to a few weeks, depending upon the nature and extent of the incurred damage.

Staying Motivated

Something that is more important than exercise itself is staying motivated to continue working out. Your initial goal to look younger and staying hotter can be a very solid reason for sticking to your plans, but other commitments and responsibilities do tend to change your priorities, which results in pushing work outs down in the list. Sometimes lack of achievement in goals too has a demoralizing effect.

To avoid this here are a few ways to stay motivated

- Plan on ways to get past obstacles *before* they happen. If you find you're skipping exercise because of family responsibilities, plan a family walk or outing to get them involved too.
- Try to work out in the mornings, you'll have more energy throughout the day and you won't have the excuse of skipping it because you're tired or have to work late.
- Workout with a friend. When a friend is waiting for you, you're less likely to back out!
- Make a list of goals and put them on the refrigerator. When you think about skipping your work out, go back and read your list. Remember why you're doing this!
- Keep track of your progress. When you reach a goal it will motivate you to keep on going.
- Wake up each day and ask yourself how you'll make your day healthy. Plan your workouts the night before and be prepared with a workout bag ready to go so there are no excuses!

⊕ Reward yourself! It's important to pat yourself on the back for reaching your goals. Get yourself a massage, a new pair of workout shoes or a night on the town every so often.

Remember life is great; you just have to feel equally great to enjoy it. That is only possible when you are in a healthy state of mind and body.

Rule #4 Indulge in Mind Activities

The fact remains that you body can feel as healthy as your mind makes it believe. This is again a fact that a healthy body carries a healthy mind, but at the same time a healthy mind is the basic requirement for a healthy body. We talk about physical exercise all the time but what about our mind.

Indeed our mind or you can say our brain needs to be exercised as much as our body needs it. To have an active brain we have to give it the sufficient quantity of the correct exercise. This will not just boost our mental faculties but helps us to stay young.

The first thing we have to know is what makes our brain active and what makes it slow down? The answer is very simple. Long unchanged routine work worries, physical and mental inactivity makes our brain dull.

No matter what you do. You need a change once in a while in order to break the monotony of the routine.

Importance of Mental Health

Job, kids, husband, home, grocery shopping and in laws are enough to drive a woman out of her mind every day. These things don't look so bad but actually they are. These little irritants keep piling up till the time a real mountain out of mole hill is created. There are numerous other reasons for which affect the mental health of a woman, some have their bases embedded in biological problems while others have their roots in the psychological domain of ailments.

What is important is the fact that women are more prone to falling prey to mental diseases, of which stroke is the most recurring. According to a recent survey in USA, the figures for middle aged women falling victim to stroke has increased from 0.5% to an alarming 2%, which is very high. The causes behind this huge increase are

⊕ Lack of exercise

⊕ Obesity

⊕ Job related stress

⊕ Insecurity on the domestic front

⊕ Inadequate or imbalanced nutrition

⊕ Lack of mental activity

⊕ Genetically inherited mental disorders

The reasons other than the genetically inherited mental disorders are all within the control of an individual who decides to do something about them, I mean you. You alone can fight back and prove not to be among the unfortunate 2%.

The only impediment is a lack of resolve. If you have decided to make yourself a better person, then there is no way that anything can affect you.

Your mental state dictates many things that would matter to not only you but will have an effect on your entire family and your community.

Studies in this field have revealed that a regular mental exercise helps in fighting off mental fatigue and depression which is caused due to stagnation of mental faculties. These exercises are not like any physical exercises but are basically aimed at regenerating your interest in life in the broader prospective.

These mental exercises are simply nothing but things that interest you in life. In order to activate your mind you are simply required to do either of the things that I have listed below.

⊕ Solve a few crossword puzzles every day.

⊕ Join a course in a subject that interests you the most.

⊕ Join a social club

⊕ Volunteer in a social activity in the field that interests you the most, provided it is not related to your job.

⊕ Help the under privileged people of the society. There is no satisfaction like the one you get from helping out someone who needs it.

⊕ Volunteer as a teacher in a school. This too is not meant for you if you are a teacher already.

⊕ Volunteer at a day care center. Little babies give a lot of satisfaction and helps keep your mind off your other problems provided you don't have your own to take care of, or you own kids have grown up and moved away.

Life is something to enjoy and the biggest thing to enjoy is the joy itself. If you have stopped enjoying yourself then it is time to stop and take a step back to see where you have messed up the things. There are chances that if you are honest with yourself you are likely to find the actual cause. It is critically important for the housewives to understand the importance of mental health and equally important for their spouses and children to realize that it is not very easy to do a job which is not always appreciated when done well but very readily the shortcomings are pointed out. To stay in a mentally fit condition, a house wife has to lay down a few rules for the other members of her family.

These may or may include your requirement of being appreciated on a regular basis but should have some or all of these included

⊕ Everything that happens or needs to get done is not your responsibility. All the members of the family must contribute in doing some of the household chores with equal responsibility.

⊕ Like all jobs, this job also requires a day off every week which does not only require the other members to agree principally but agree to follow in true spirit.

⊕ If not on daily basis but at least once a week you need to get out of your work place for some peace and quiet preferably without the other members. For this you can arrange an evening with your friends.

⊕ Every day you need some time off for yourself which should be purely your own time during which you can pursue you physical fitness regime and your social activities.

Breaking the vicious circle of routine is very important for everyone. Those who get stuck in it are the ones who end up in a wreck. These tips mentioned above are basically required to break the monotony in your life. That will take your mind off the daily routine problems and will give you the required break.

The working women have a set of problems of their own. These are no less complicated than those of the housewives.

They have to juggle to different environments, office and home at the same time. For the singles it has a different set of problems and for those with a family responsibility, the problems are different in nature. In all the cases the girl has to survive while handling her professional and domestic life at the same time, with very less time to pamper herself to the extent she deserves. Let me make one thing absolutely clear. In this world there is no other person who can take better care of you than yourself.

If you have decided to neglect yourself, then others will follow suit.

For the professional lady the time constraints are much higher than those on a housewife. She has deadlines to meet at both the work and home front. This is enough mental load on a person to forget about looking pretty and feeling good. What here is important is that you reassess your stance and work out a plan for yourself to give yourself a timeout from your routine, just for your mental health. What I have mentioned earlier is the way to break your monotonous routine of responsibilities and give some time to yourself.

Your requirement for mental exercise is as much needed as by the housewives, or maybe more. The reason is restricted application of mental faculties, both at work place and at home. It may not be true for all as regards to work place but at home there is only stagnation. You also need to create a world outside your routine life.

Agility, activity and alertness are what you need to revive that lost vitality in your life. What you have to do is get time for yourself.

Lots of women in their middle age go through a crisis just trying to find their own selves in the hassle and bustle of every day routine. They find the mom making breakfast before she goes to work. She finds the pet owner at the vet's. She finds the occasional lover of her spouse too, but who she fails to find is her own self. This creates a lot of confusion in her subconscious mind. This may not be evident or maybe you don't even find it applicable to you, but try locating your own identity, not related through others. This will make you realize your actual problem.

As a matter of fact this is just a mental conflict which actually does not have an issue that would drive anyone to the loony bin, but to resolve this issue does help you in making many decisions and at a later stage in life where clarity of mind is more important than anything else.

You must focus yourself to understand that by reading this book and then following it, you will not shed off twenty years of your age from your appearance or look cool trying to frolic like a teenage girl, but what I intend here is to teach you that whatever your age maybe, late 30's, 40, 50 or 60, you can live your life to the fullest.

This can only be achieved if you have a sound mind and a sound body which is only possible if you have control over your situation. That only is possible when you are already in a position or are already making your own decisions.

This only comes with practice. When it comes to decision making, our mind starts responding in a particularly trained fashion with passage of time as a habit. You automatically start buying clothes of almost the same style when you go for buying clothes for work.

Your choice almost becomes the same when it comes to selection of a formal dress. Even there is no real variety in your choice of food or vacation. Everything is automatic.

This becomes the comfort zone for many, but this tends to stop the brain from exercising its self. That is where stagnation comes. There is an old saying, "What does not advance must retrograde".

It is very true, when it comes to us, we actually stop being youthful and aging takes over. In order to defeat aging we have to keep advancing with youthful fervor to continue being young at heart.

For this we have to maintain our individuality and keep exercising our mind by adopting out of routine activities which I have mentioned earlier. Those should not be taken as a final authority; you are a free person to choose for yourself what makes you happy and gives you a feeling of fulfillment. Just do it and feel good about it.

Rule #5 Move Around Be Social

"The biggest education is not from the books, it is from the people you meet. I know more, for I meet more people and learn for them, every single day".

For me friends are like an insurance policy, which comes in handy whenever you need them. More the merrier, these terms are time tested and are good for all ages.

There is no restriction on age to make new friends. As a matter of fact, those friends that you make at a mature age are the ones who really are compatible with you.

As we age it becomes our tendency to remain attaches to things and people who we are well conversant with over a period of time. This makes our circle of friends limited. The input we get from our social circle is also limited, without any variety. Same old topics to discuss!

The same old problems keep popping up again and again. You don't even feel like dressing up when you are with them, the homely bunch, as someone refers to them, they have already seen you in the best and the worst, so it hardly makes any difference. The actual difference lies not in what they have seen or not, but rather in your attitude, the middle aged attitude.

If you desire to feel younger again get out of the house and move around. Make new friends and acquaintances. How is this possible? That is very simple. Join a class or a club which you always wanted to, but never got the chance or time earlier.

You will be surprised to find out that most of the people there have almost similar ideas as yours with little variation and lots of new thing for you to learn, besides the subject itself. The reason is that, it was what you wanted to do and so do they. That is the first common between you and them.

Moving further, chances are that you might catch up with life and youth from where you left it and boarded the middle aged express, which I can tell you very safely that it doesn't take you anywhere but to a retirement home after a very tiring journey.

New people bring new ideas and new society. In some cases altogether a new way of life for you, with a promise of an opportunity to explore more of this world, altogether with a new vision.

This is likely to give your mind the much needed exercise that we have discussed earlier.

Benefits of Joining a Fitness Club

Joining a fitness club definitely has its advantages than joining any other club or community group. The positive thing is that all the benefits are directly for you. Here are a few of those that I have jotted down for you.

⊕ The club helps you to get back in shape and makes you get back the strength and vigor that you need.

⊕ You get to meet new people with a lot of experience in health and physical fitness who are old members of that club.

⊕ You are likely to get good health tips from the experienced ones.

⊕ Availability of personal trainer ensures proper and systematic physical training for you.

⊕ Getting into a friendly competition with other members will of the club can be fun and rewarding for you in the long run.

⊕ Being in the club is itself sufficient motivation to keep up your progress.

Benefits of Joining a Social Club

Social clubs offer a lot of opportunities to its members. The most important feature which I feel, that these clubs offer is the opportunity to meet other people. I strongly believe that meeting people is a great way to enhance your life. What we can derive from these meetings is an altogether a new outlook towards life itself.

We all have our own experiences to get guidance from, but at the same time we can enhance our knowledge from the experiences of others. New ideas and new concepts make us better than before. This is what life is all about, meeting people and making friends. Who knows that your soul mate might be lurking around there waiting to meet you?

Benefits of Joining a Class

When they say, "You can't teach old dog new tricks" it is only good when applied to an old dog. You are not a dog. Remember, you are God's best creation ever. It is never too late to learn a new trick or two. So go ahead, join a class. It really is good for you. Just think what you always wanted to do. It can be anything, dancing, music, cooking, computers and accounting or for that matter creative writing, just think and join it. You will realize what you had been missing all along. These classes give you a new thing to work up on, meaning that you will be involved in something new. Try not to join an advanced class. A basic class for the beginners would be ideal, especially in the field which you had no previous knowledge or you had dropped out in the initial stage for some reason would be a great idea.

Even though this may not give you a profession to pursue in the future, but will give you enough to pursue a hobby. The benefits that it will give you are tremendous. Your mind will exercise in another direction giving you enough mental occupation that your routine worries will be long over with. You might find answers to some of your problems as it happens in many cases, when you venture in another direction you are likely to solve certain outstanding issues.

Conclusion

A 104 year old Japanese woman and mother of 11 kids, was asked once that to what factor does she owe her long life to? Her reply was "I owe my long life to the fact that I didn't die young". This is one way of dealing with what you have and the other is to make worthwhile of what you have. Life is a very precious thing. To protect it and to keep it in the best possible way is everyone's duty.

It is very important to understand that life is totally dependent on balance. This balance is required in every field of our lives. Starting from sleeping, eating and playing to learning and making friends, all things need to be balanced. Deficiency in one aspect cannot be covered with excess in another.

What we do in life is called compromise and in no way can be called living.

Youth is the state of mind which liberated us from the social taboos and allows us to live as we feel please with strength and vigor. That is what makes youth so desirable. With age come social inhabitations and limitations. We tend to tie ourselves down with social norms and self imposed bans.

To fight out with this state of mind, it is required that we have the physical strength and mental ability. After a certain age it can only be acquired with a lot of effort.

This effort has to be in the correct direction to maintain our body and mind which is only possible when we make good use of our body and provide it with the best that it requires, that is balanced diet and sufficient exercise. The most important is the correct attitude. Your correct attitude can cover up your physical and aptitude deficiencies in any field of life.

This gets us back what we call youth, with its vigor, strength and desire to be someone and the desire to live this beautiful life which can only be enjoyed with youth.

I wish all my readers to have a healthy and prosperous life, with everlasting youth.

"God Bless to all My Family & Friends. You are always in my prayers whether I tell you daily or not"

Harry J. Misner

FREE BONUS

Once my new author website is finished being designed, everyone who purchases any of my books will be granted lifetime access using the login information below:

http://www.harrymisner.com/books

Username: customer

Password: appreciation

Here you'll be able to ask me any questions you might have via email and purchase updated or additional books & eBooks of mine at a discounted rate.

Dedication: I dedicate this book to my beautiful son Collin, who just turned 3 years old this September and is currently battling Autism. I constantly call him my little Angel, because he has changed my life more than I've ever dreamed or imagined possible.

I love you buddy!

"Today, 1 in 150 individuals are diagnosed with autism, making it more common than pediatric cancer, diabetes, and AIDS combined."

So please help the fight, visit http://www.autismspeaks.org/

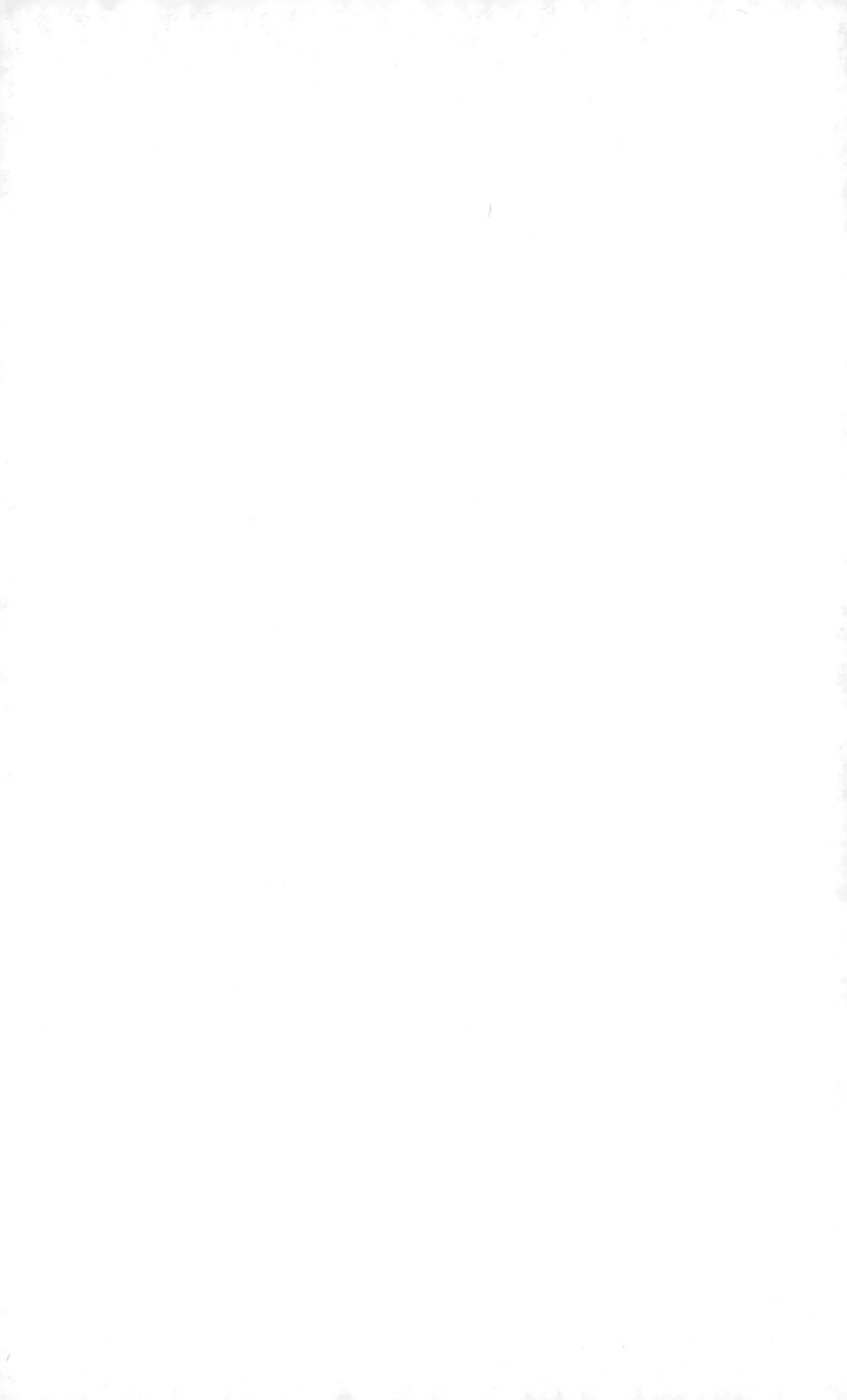

www.ingramcontent.com/pod-product-compliance
Lightning Source LLC
Chambersburg PA
CBHW060635290526
45793CB00001B/264